SENSUAL MASSAGE

The Joy of Touch

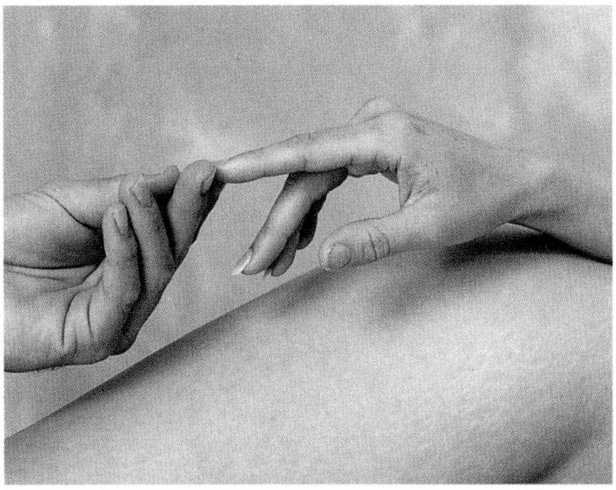